Made in United States
Troutdale, OR
11/03/2024

24410956R00058